TAKE WOMEN TO ORGASM

TRY THESE THINGS YOUR WOMAN WILL NEVER LEAVE YOU

BY

MATHEW J. ASHTON

TABLE OF CONTENTS

INTRODUCTION

Can we just be real for a minute, numerous ladies have never experienced climax and a large number of them won't ever will! The purposes behind this change, yet the most widely recognized among them, has to do with the man, or men by and large, that they are having intercourse with.

You could ponder and inquire as to why climax is so critical to ladies and a similar inquiry can be posed to why it means a lot to men. On the off chance that you don't have any idea, as a man, when discharge, or cum or delivery - whichever one you need to call it - that is you, as a man, hitting your climax; and it is significantly more simpler for men to arrive at that peak than it is for ladies. To that end ladies discuss climax - or an absence of it - more frequently than you would presumably need to hear.

In any case, in decency, it is generally challenging for some ladies to peak through penetrative sex; to that end you see bunches of ladies encountering climax just when they jerk off - and that is on the grounds that they can contact the delicate pieces of their vagina which thus makes them arrive at joyous beyond words. Sadly, relatively few people know this, consequently, they simply focus on entrance and their own climax.

In this book you will find all the data you really want, along alongside the tips and procedures to appreciate sex and cause your accomplice to appreciate it as well. Abandon your feelings of dread and your questions!

What's more, try to know the approaches to a climax and joy.

SECTION 1

FEMALE ORGASMS

Female climaxes: What you want to be aware

Dissimilar to certain creatures, human females can have intercourse any time, and they don't need to climax to ovulate or get pregnant.

Male-overwhelmed logical standards imply that much about the female climax stays misconstrued, and numerous unsafe legends endure.

A female climax can be profoundly pleasurable and happen during masturbation or sexual action with at least one accomplices. Researchers are uncertain whether it has extra advantages.

In this article, we take a gander at why female climaxes happen and what occurs during a climax. We additionally expose a few normal misguided judgments.

FOR WHAT REASON DO FEMALES ORGASMS?

A climax can cause extraordinary joy, which might have its own advantages.
The advantages of the male climax are clear. Men should discharge to store sperm in the vagina, perhaps prompting pregnancy. The male climax, thusly, fills an unmistakable developmental need.

The motivation behind the female climax is less clear. Analysts have proposed various likely advantages, however few have been thoroughly tried, and no hypothesis has decisive logical help.

Not all that the body does has an unmistakable reason, in any case. Researchers have not found the developmental advantages of certain qualities that have continued in people.

A 2016 studyTrusted Source contends that the female climax might have no conspicuous transformative advantage and that it could be a remnant of when the chemicals related with climax were important for a lady to ovulate.

Since there was no developmental need to take out the female climax, it persevered in any event, when it was presently excessive for ripeness.

Climax might fill significant needs, nonetheless. The delight it can cause can urge females to engage in sexual relations. This may likewise advance holding with a sexual accomplice, which has critical transformative advantages.

WHAT HAPPENS DURING AN ORGASM?

During excitement, bloodstream to the privates increments, making them become more delicate.

As excitement builds, an individual's pulse, circulatory strain, and breathing rate may likewise increment. As the climax draws near, the muscles might jerk or fit. Numerous ladies experience musical muscle fits in the vagina during a climax.

A few scientists have suggested that sexual reaction follows explicit stages, however their speculations about these stages contrast.

In any case, most hypotheses incorporate the accompanying stages:

- fervor, during which excitement constructs
- level, during which excitement increments and levels off
- climax, which causes serious sensations of delight

- goal, during which excitement decreases

Numerous females can have one more climax after goal, though guys ordinarily require a time of rest prior to having another climax.

MEDICAL ADVANTAGES

While the web is loaded up with articles promising that climaxes further develop skin, hair, and in general wellbeing, there is minimal logical proof that climaxes offer a particular medical advantage.

Researchers have not recognized any transformative advantages of female climaxes or found that climaxes further develop wellbeing.

However, climaxes are pleasurable, and delight can be its own advantage. Pleasurable sex might work on an individual's state of mind, ease pressure, help insusceptibility, and encourage better connections.

Ladies don't have to climax to get pregnant. Nonetheless, a restricted collection of proof proposes that climaxes might support ripeness.

One tiny studyTrusted Source, for instance, estimated whether there was better sperm maintenance after female climax. While the outcomes affirmed this, demonstrating that the female body holds sperm better after a climax will require bigger examinations with plans of better caliber.

NORMAL MISCONCEPTIONS

Individuals hold numerous misguided judgments about female climaxes. A few legends include:

1. Ladies who might climax at any point have mental issues.

While injury, relationship issues, and poor mental healthTrusted Source can make it more challenging to climax, many individuals with solid sexual perspectives great connections actually experience issues.

A climax is both a physical and mental reaction, and various medical conditions can make it more hard to appreciate sex along these lines.

Certain individuals battle to climax because of lacking oil. This might occur while taking hormonal conception prevention, or during or after pregnancy, or because of menopause.

Likewise, ladies can encounter vulvodynia, which alludes to unexplained agony in the vagina or around the vulva. Treating this and other ailments might work on sexual delight.

2. Climaxes from penetrative sex are normal or the best type of sexual articulation.

Self-selected specialists, generally men, have long let ladies know that they should climax from hetero intercourse. Nonetheless, numerous ladies can climax from clitoral feeling.

Sigmund FreudTrusted Source contended that the vaginal climax was the predominant and more full grown climax. No proof backings this case.

3. Ladies can't have vaginal climaxes.

While vaginal climaxes are more uncommon than those from clitoral excitement, a few ladies have them — regardless of other feelings.

The female climax can result from many kinds of feeling, including vaginal, clitoral, and areola contact.

Not every person climaxes from a similar sort of feeling.

Ladies should be infatuated to climax.

Climax is a complex mental and natural experience — coming to and encountering climax isn't something very similar for each lady. A few ladies might have to feel love to climax, while others may not.

An individual's relationship with their accomplice could possibly impact their capacity to climax during sex.

A 2018 studyTrusted Source discovered that 86% of lesbian ladies said they normally or consistently climax during sex, contrasted with only 66% of sexually unbiased ladies and 65% of hetero ladies.

Members were bound to climax oftentimes on the off chance that they:

- gotten more oral sex
- had longer-enduring sex
- announced higher relationship fulfillment
- requested what they needed in bed
- taken part in sexual messages or calls
- communicated love during sex
- carried on sexual dreams

- attempted new sexual positions

4. An accomplice can determine whether a lady has had a climax.

It is basically impossible to know if a lady has had a climax without asking her. Certain individuals make commotions during a climax, while others are quiet. Some flush or sweat after a climax, yet others don't.

An individual who wants to find out whether their accomplice has had a climax can ask without being fierce.

In the event that the response is no, stay away from judgment, outrage, or insecurities — these can come down on the individual to climax, which can prompt uneasiness and make it more troublesome. All things being equal, examine whether they would favor an alternate way to deal with sex.

IMAGINE A SCENARIO IN WHICH YOU CAN'T ORGASM.

Being not able to climax is a typical issue, and it can happen for different reasons. Certain individuals may not get the right sort of feeling during sex, while others might have encountered injury connected to sex. Others may just be uninterested.

A 2018 analysisTrusted Source of 135 earlier investigations recognized a few factors that increment the gamble of sexual brokenness, including:

- relationship issues
- stress
- psychological wellness issues
- poor actual wellbeing
- genitourinary issues, like pelvic agony
- a background marked by fetus removal
- a past filled with female genital mutilation
- sexual maltreatment
- being strict, maybe because of sexual disgrace and shame

A similar report distinguished a few modifiable gamble factors that work on sexual experience, including:

- work out
- day to day love from an accomplice
- a positive self-perception
- sex training
- close correspondence with an accomplice

Masturbation can assist an individual with finding what feels significantly better to them. A few different systems that could help include:

- utilizing sexual greases to make sex more agreeable
- requesting that an accomplice invigorate the clitoris during sex
- jerking off during sex
- examining dreams with an accomplice
- telling an accomplice on the off chance that something doesn't feel much better

The previously mentioned 2018 studyTrusted Source.that thought about climax recurrence among individuals of different sexual directions in the United States found that the accompanying ways of behaving during sex improve the probability of ladies having a climax:

- profound kissing
- genital feeling during vaginal intercourse
- oral sex
- In the event that self improvement procedures don't work, a specialist who has practical experience in sexual brokenness might have the option to recognize an issue, assuming there is one.

Take A climax troublesome, including:

- an absence of oil
- hormonal irregular characteristics
- pelvic torment
- muscle brokenness
- a past filled with injury

At the point when injury or relationship issues make having a climax troublesome, or when an individual feels embarrassed about sex or their longings, individual or couples guiding can help.

DISORDERS

Orgasmic issues can prompt pain, disappointment, and sensations of disgrace, both for the individual encountering the side effects and their sexual accomplice.

In spite of the fact that climaxes happen in much the same way in all sexes, medical care experts will generally portray climax problems in gendered terms.

FEMALE ORGASMIC DISORDERS

Female orgasmic messes are based on the nonappearance or huge deferral of climaxes following adequate excitement.

Specialists allude to the shortfall of having climaxes as anorgasmia. This term can either allude to when an individual has never experiencedTrusted Source a climax (essential anorgasmia) or when an individual who recently experienced climaxes never again can (optional anorgasmia). The condition can happen by and large or in unambiguous circumstances.

Female orgasmic issues can happen as the aftereffect of actual causes, like gynecological circumstances or the utilization of specific meds, or mental causes like uneasiness or sorrow.

SECTION 2

THE CLITORIS

The clitoris: What is there to be aware of this secret organ?
That most subtle piece of the female life structures: the clitoris. What is it, where is it found, and how can it respond? How could it be created, and for what reason don't we hear a lot about it? We answer this large number of inquiries and more in this Spotlight.
The clitoris has for some time been distorted and misconstrued, and even now, it actually holds a few enigmas that science is yet to settle.

Every single female warm blooded creature — and a few female birds and reptiles — have a clitoris (or two, just like with snakes).

In any case, it isn't clear if or the number of them additionally climax thanks to this organ.

In people, the clitoris has been solidly attached to sexual delight, however whether it assumes some other part is as yet a matter for banter.

Regardless of roughly a portion of the total populace being brought into the world with a clitoris, this sexual organ isn't discussed definitely, and, until as of late, even the data that we could have found about it in course readings was erroneous or deceiving.

Anyway, what could have been some significant awareness of this slippery organ, and for what reason would we say we are as yet attempting to grasp it? Peruse on to find out.

1. MORE THAN JUST A 'LITTLE HILL'

The idea of the clitoris can be tracked down in the actual name; "clitoris" comes from the Ancient Greek word "kleitorisTrusted Source," signifying "little slope," and which itself may likewise be connected with "kleis," signifying "key."

Albeit this organ might be the key that opens female sexual joy, it isn't only a bit of "slope," as it has for some time been accepted.

Truth be told, the little slope (safeguarded by a shroud of skin, or the "clitoral hood," which is viewed as over the urethral opening) is only the tip of a much bigger organ that is the clitoris.

That tip, called the clitoral organ, is the most promptly apparent piece of this genital organ.

However the whole organ expands a lot farther than that, and this thought was at first brought to public consideration a couple of years prior by specialist Dr. Helen O'Connell.

"The vaginal wall is, truth be told, the clitoris. On the off chance that you lift the skin off the vagina as an afterthought walls, you get the bulbs of the clitoris — three-sided, crescent masses of erectile tissue,"

The clitoris has three significant parts:

- The glans clitoris, which is the main noticeable piece of the organ, representing "a fifth or less" of the whole construction

- the two crura, which expand, similar to sections, down from the glans clitoris and profound into the tissue of the vulva, on one or the other side
- the two bulbs of the vestibule, which broaden either side of the vaginal opening (not all specialists concur that the vestibular bulbs have a connection to the clitoris, nonetheless; scientists Vincenzo and Giulia Puppo, for example, argueTrusted Source that the clitoris comprises "of the glans, body, and crura" as it were)

Completely, the clitoris might reach upwards of 7 centimeters long, while perhaps not longer, and the glans makes up around 4-7 millimeters of the entirety.

The glans is likewise the part that is most extravagant in free sensitive spots, hence giving the most sensation.

2. 'GREAT CENTRAL STATION OF EROTIC SENSATION'

Because of its elevated degree of responsiveness, the clitoris is typically the principal player with regards to the female climax.

Mainstream society and obscene material frequently will quite often portray the female climax as something normally feasible exclusively through infiltration, however science recounts an alternate story out and out.

Most ladies, scientists have found, will possibly accomplish climax when the clitoris — or, all the more explicitly, the glans clitoris — is additionally animated.

As a matter of fact, ongoing investigations recommend that ladies who experience the more uncommon, and at times more questionable kinds of climax — vaginal climax because of infiltration, or vaginal climax through G spot excitement — may really have clitoral feelings to thank.

3. A FEMALE PENIS?

The clitoris has likewise in some cases been viewed as a female penis, generally because of a peculiarity that we might allude to as "natural homology," which alludes to the way that all hatchlings are conceived, as Emily Nagoski puts it, with "overall similar part, coordinated in various ways."

This is likewise why men — who, in contrast to ladies, won't require, or be capable, to communicate milk and bosom feed children — have areolas.

They actually foster areolas, notwithstanding, on the grounds that they — like essentially all body parts — are prearranged in the earliest phases of undeveloped turn of events.

At the end of the day, people really reflect each other physiologically to an extremely incredible degree.

Furthermore, this is the way the clitoris creates; it and the penis are homologues.

4. DEVELOPMENTAL RELIC OR EROTIC BONUS?

While the penis and the clitoris are homologous, in any case, the penis assumes a few parts — sensual, regenerative, and excretive — while the clitoris performs just a single work: that of causing sexual situation, which might prompt climax. For what reason could that be? However, a few specialists accept that the female climax may not necessarily in all cases have been "a reward."

All things being equal, that's what they feel, corresponding to male climax — which harmonizes with the arrival of semen — female climax might have animated the arrival of ovules.
In any case, the substances in this way delivered in the body, the researchers say, are similar to those delivered in the collections of other female warm blooded animals, for example, rodents during intercourse, animating the arrival of eggs that can be prepared.

In people, ovulation is an unconstrained occasion, free from intercourse. However, the creators of the previously mentioned study guess that, sooner or later in our transformative past, we might well have worked like different vertebrates, and female climax might have animated the arrival of ovules.

Presently, climax has continued as a pleasurable transformative inheritance, without the conceptive affiliation.

5. WHY IS THE CLITORIS SO TABOO?

However, why has it taken such a long time for researchers to begin taking a greater amount of an interest in the clitoris, and how can it be that somebody just stepped up to the plate and outputted the clitoris and produced an exact portrayal of it in 2009?

No one got a kick out of the chance to discuss it, and the issue, the specialists recommended, began in the home.

They state, "[B]ecause the clitoris' just capability is for sexual delight, guardians have no […] motivation to examine the clitoris."

All the more amazingly, however, they found, "Even 'specialists' giving exhortation to guardians have utilized terms other than clitoris" while talking about the significance of female genitalia.

In a culture that has zeroed in on the significance of multiplication to the impediment of happiness, the clitoris has lain neglected, and the general population and clinical experts the same have felt humiliated to examine and focus harder on it.

However the absence of a discussion about female genitalia and female joy might influence the manner by which ladies grasp their sexual wellbeing, and it might try and effect their sexual experiences.

"Recovering the clitoris might assist women with effectively finding their own sexual delight and be more free in that their sexual decisions," close Ogletree and Ginsburg.

We trust that this Spotlight can advance the discussion about the clitoris, and that it has furnished you with additional knowledge into the marvels of female sexuality.

TRY THESE THINGS YOUR WOMAN WILL NEVER LEAVE YOU

Can we just be real for a minute, numerous ladies have never experienced climax and a large number of them won't ever will! The explanations behind this fluctuate, yet the most widely recognized among them has to do withe man, or men by and large, that they are engaging in sexual relations with.

You could ponder and inquire as to why climax is so vital to ladies and a similar inquiry can be posed to why it means a lot to men. On the off chance that you don't have the foggiest idea, as a man, when discharge, or cum or delivery - whichever one you need to call it - that is you, as a man, hitting your climax; and it is considerably more simpler for men to arrive at that peak than it is for ladies. To that end ladies discuss climax - or an absence of it - more frequently than you would most likely need to hear.

Yet, in decency, it is generally challenging for some ladies to peak through penetrative sex; to that end you see bunches of ladies encountering climax just when they stroke off - and that is on the grounds that they can contact the delicate

pieces of their vagina which thusly makes them arrive at beyond happy. Sadly, very few people know this, thus, they simply focus on infiltration and their own climax.
However, today, I will give you hints that will assist you with turning into a superman in bed and make her peak however much as could reasonably be expected.

- TRY NOT TO RUSH HER VAGINA

This might sound in opposition to what you ought to do yet believe me, you would rather not center too early around her vagina. Reality you likely don't know is that ladies love to have their entire body investigated first prior to getting down there. Be that as it may, numerous men are excessively fixated on getting in straight and hurry to the vagina, when she is anticipating that you should go through her body. You want not to be in a hurry, find an opportunity to investigate her body to set her in the mind-set for what is to come eventually. Continuously recall that the vagina is typically the end, not the start. Take it easy, don't rush it .

- OPENNESS IS ABSOLUTELY VITAL

Quite possibly of the greatest slip-up couples make - and not simply men now - is their inability to impart their sexual necessities to one another. You genuinely should discuss your sexual necessities with your accomplice, and furthermore have them impart theirs to you. For men, this assists you with understanding her body better, and what she is in all likelihood going to answer. For ladies, imparting your sexual sentiments and necessities to your man is significant. Try not to expect they should understand what you need, no. You need to let them know what you need and how you need. Assuming that you are old and striking to the point of having intercourse, you ought to be old and intense enough to discuss it.

This follows the correspondence part. As well as imparting, it is essential to permit her to start to lead the pack since she really wants the experience and should be satisfied. As a man, you need to humor her in this and cause her to feel exceptional by permitting her to start to lead the pack in what she needs from you in bed.

Sex specialist Ian Kerner, Ph.D., LMFT, says that utilizing your mouth is the most ideal way to get a feeling of what your accomplice likes at each phase of excitement, including the stage not long before climax. You'll realize your accomplice is turning out to be more stimulated on the off chance that you notice expanded vaginal oil or on the other hand assuming the outer part of their clitoris or their whole vulva grows. The clitoris — including the wishbone-formed segment that is under the skin — is made of erectile tissue very much like the penis, so assuming your accomplice's private parts expand in size, you're working effectively! To figure out additional about your accomplice's inclinations, let them start to lead the pack. While you're giving them oral sex, get between their legs and provide them with a strong base of lips, tongue, and even jawline (on the off chance that you have a perfect, smooth shave, that is) to rub against. While your accomplice does the crushing, note how hard they're pushing and in what bearing. Utilize that data some other time while utilizing your fingers or mouth to satisfy them.

- TRY NOT TO RACE TOWARD YOUR PARTNER'S ORGASM.

"Attempt to recollect the objective of sex is joy, and climax is one sort of delight that is altogether more limited than the remainder of it. Take as much time as necessary with your developments, and don't zero in on the final plan. There is a slight incongruity to it — the more your accomplice contemplates climaxing, the more outlandish they will be to climax. So ease the heat off of your accomplice and spotlight on causing them to feel better as workable as far as might be feasible. (We allude to this stoppage method as shutting the "delight hole.")

- CONSOLIDATE EXTERNAL CLITORAL STIMULATION.

Priorities straight: by far most of vulva-proprietors require outer clitoral excitement to arrive at climax. Truth be told, an investigation of in excess of 1,000 vulva-proprietors in 2017 uncovered that just 18% of members could climax through vaginal intercourse alone. So while you're engaging in sexual relations, you need to zero in on outside excitement alone or in mix with some type of entrance.

If you have any desire to animate your accomplice's clitoris during P-in-V intercourse, some sex positions make it more straightforward to do than others. Rachel* I really love the coital arrangement method, or CAT: "When a person is on top of you in the evangelist position, have him shift his body somewhat forward so that, each time he pushes, his penis rubs against your clitoris." This strategy is significantly more orgasmic assuming your accomplice's legs are together and you're riding them, says Ellen Friedrichs, M.A., a wellbeing teacher who likewise teaches at the City University of New York's City Tech grounds. You can accomplish a similar impact when they're on top by setting yourself up on your elbows, which puts your midsection in nearer contact with their clitoris.

- FOCUS CLOSER ON THEIR BUTT.

Except if butt-centric is on the menu, butts are ordinarily sidelined during sex. Furthermore, that is a disgrace, on the grounds that "the bottom are loaded with sensitive spots," says Gilda Carle, Ph.D., a universally known relationship master. To give your accomplice "an astounding shock of delight," spread your fingers wide and press their cheeks.
All things considered, you ought to inquire as to whether they're into goods crushing first. In the event that they're down, be delicate, and approach it slowly and carefully. Indeed, obviously, there are individuals out there who pine for a decent, hard hitting, however that should be examined and settled on before the butt smacking starts.

- TRY NOT TO STOP KISSING THEM.

When things get more warmed, you may be enticed to zero in less on kissing for additional X-appraised joys. Yet, profound kissing is frequently an unquestionable necessity for arriving at climax, as per a 2017 review of in excess of 50,000 grown-ups. The discoveries uncovered that vulva-proprietors were significantly more liable to arrive at climax assuming that their sexual experience incorporated a mix of profound kissing, oral sex, and genital feeling.

- ENJOY THEIR FANTASIES.

Inquire as to whether they have any dreams they might want to investigate. "Dreams can increment excitement during a sexual encounter," says Francis. "Finding a dream that truly turns your accomplice on can add one more layer of delight during sex." It's likewise a method for getting your accomplice all the more mentally excited, which is similarly as significant (while possibly not more significant) than actual excitement with regards to having a climax. One investigation discovered that vulva-proprietors with lower sexual craving will more often than not need mental excitement to perceive their actual excitement. Attempt pretend or recount to your accomplice a suggestive story to kick their pleasure up a score.

- SPEAK PROFANELY TO THEM.

"Filthy talk" doesn't need to incorporate four-letter words. Depict how you're treating your accomplice, or express out loud whatever you believe they should do to you. In the event that you're reluctant, a straightforward commendation about how appealing you find your accomplice will get the job done. "Offering something explicit about me is provocative while we're sleeping," says Emily*. Furthermore, assuming your accomplice has let you know ahead of time that they're turned on by unambiguous words and expressions, pepper those into the exchange, as well.

- LUBE UP.

Regardless of how hot and weighty you're getting, without satisfactory oil, it's simple for sex to become awkward or even difficult for your accomplice. While lube is totally essential for butt-centric sex (butts don't self-grease up like vaginas do), it's useful for vaginal infiltration and outside feeling, as well. "Grease expands the solace and speed with which you can infiltrate the vagina and grate against the clitoris," says Friedrichs.

Recollect that requiring lube doesn't mean your accomplice isn't turned on — a few bodies simply get wetter than others. Furthermore, medicine, hormonal irregular characteristics, menopause, stress, and parchedness can all diminish the body's regular grease, so nothing bad can be said about requiring some extra tricky stuff. Utilizing lube makes sex more agreeable for all interested parties. As a matter of fact, a recent report found that utilizing lube improves sexual joy for vulva-proprietors. That's simply recollecting whether you're utilizing condoms, you ought to stay with water-based or silicone-based lube, since oil-based lube can harm plastic.

- CENTER AROUND THEIR NECK.

Our necks are exceptionally responsive touch cushions: the skin is meager there, and the veins are near the surface. So it's not shocking that analysts have observed that the neck is one of the most outstanding spots for feeling utilizing light touch (so no hickeys, please — except if your accomplice requests one).
While you're engaging in sexual relations and your accomplice is obviously pushing toward climax, brush your lips from their collarbone to their jaw, then, at that point, give their neck delicate, warm kisses to drive them wild.

- BREAK OUT THE SEX TOYS.

You can't construct a house without a mallet, and for some vulva-proprietors, you can't fabricate a climax without a vibrator. Over half of vulva-proprietors use vibrators to assist them with accomplishing climax, as indicated by a recent report, so inviting delight devices into the room ought to be an easy decision. Assuming you actually need persuading, a recent report found that vulva-proprietors who utilized vibrators both alone and with an accomplice revealed more noteworthy sexual fulfillment contrasted with the individuals who just utilized a vibrator without anyone else. Presently would you say you are prepared to venture into your accomplice's bedside cabinet?

Allow your accomplice to hold a vibrator against their clitoris while you infiltrate them with a dildo, your fingers, or penis; or work the toy yourself. Simply make sure to get some information about their strain and speed inclinations: you would rather not get too quick and weighty right away.

CONCLUSION

Albeit the examination of regular history proposes that climax comes from the release components of gametes, its ongoing transformative importance in vertebrates would prefer to get from post-copulatory specific systems. Climax has its starting point in the development of treatment designs, however the orgasmic signal involves a positive encounter, which underscores the outcome of the relationship. The climax could find its ongoing developmental importance in the inclination of an irrelevant sexual accomplice, in species utilizing interior preparation. Regardless, climax has normally a social support impact of contraceptive exercises.

www.ingramcontent.com/pod-product-compliance
Lightning Source LLC
LaVergne TN
LVHW020524160826
845677LV00015B/3894

* 9 7 9 8 8 4 8 0 1 4 7 5 4 *